Copyright © 2020 Laura Summers

All rights reserved. No part of this publication may be reproduced, distributed, or transmitted in any form or by any means, including photocopying, recording, or other electronic or mechanical methods, without the prior written permission of the publisher, except in the case of brief quotations embodied in critical reviews and certain other noncommercial uses permitted by copyright law.

Table of Contents

INTRODUCTION 5

    Foods to Avoid 7

    Choosing a Pancreatitis Diet 8

    Sample Menu 10

RECIPES 12

    BANANA YOGURT POTS 12

    CANNELLINI BEAN SALAD 13

    MOUSSAKA 14

    TOMATO AND WATERMELON SALAD 16

    EDGY VEGGIE WRAPS 18

    SPICY TOMATO BAKED EGGS 20

    BLUEBERRY OATS BOWL 22

    CARROT, ORANGE AND AVOCADO SALAD 24

    SALMON WITH POTATOES AND CORN SALAD 25

    MIXED BEAN SALAD 27

    SPICED CARROT AND LENTIL SOUP 29

    PANZANELLE SALAD 31

    MED CHICKEN, QUINOA AND GREEK SALAD 33

QUINOA AND STIR FRIED VEG 35

GRILLED VEGETABLE WITH BEAN MASH 37

MOROCCAN CHICKPEA SOUP 39

SPICY MEDITERRANEAN BEET SALAD 41

APPLE BUTTERNUT SQUASH PANCAKES 43

PASTIERA (PASTA EGG BAKE) 46

THANKSGIVING MEATBALLS 48

MAPLE GREEN BEANS 51

CARROT PURÉE WITH OLIVE OIL AND CILANTRO
.... 53

HEARTY VEGETABLE AND LENTIL SOUP 56

TURKEY MEATLOAF (MINI) 58

SWEET POTATO AND WHITE BEAN FRITTERS 61

RICE PUDDING 64

BANANA BLUEBERRY MUFFINS 67

BAKED BERRY FRENCH TOAST 69

PUMPKIN OATMEAL BARS 71

ASPARAGUS FRITTATA 74

VEGETABLE POPOVER 76

- EDAMAME HUMMUS WRAP 78
- SALMON BURGER WITH BOK CHOY, GINGER AND LEMONGRASS 81
- PEACHES AND CREAM SMOOTHIE 84
- TURKEY SWEET POTATO HASH 86
- TURKEY TORTELLINI SOUP 89
- VEGETABLE POPOVER 94
- CHICKEN WITH QUINOA 96
- CHICKEN KEBAB WITH TZATZIKI AND PITA 98
- CHICKEN SALAD SANDWICH 101
- SUMMER VEGETABLES OMELET 103
- SHRIMP POMODORO & ANGEL HAIR 105

INTRODUCTION

Pancreatitis occurs when the pancreas that produces your digestive enzymes becomes inflamed. The pancreas produces insulin and digestive enzymes, but these enzymes may end irritating the organ itself. This irritation may stop the pancreas from performing its function and this condition is called pancreatitis. Because of the close nature of the pancreas and the digestive system, what you choose to eat can have a major effect. Although pancreatitis inflammation is often caused by gallstones, chronic pancreatitis is even more closely related to your day-to-day diet. This book will cover everything you need to know about following a diet to help with pancreatitis, recipes and offer a sample 7 day plan to follow.

In a nutshell, a pancreas-friendly diet contains lots of protein from lean meats and contains little animal fat or simple sugars. This means you should get the majority of your protein sources from poultry, seafood and low-fat dairy. If you eat red meats, make sure you get lean meats with reduced saturated fat. These foods should make up the majority of your meals:

- Dairy – low-fat cheeses like feta and mozzarella, low-fat milk and yogurt, eggs
- Fruits and vegetables – all kinds of fruit and veg. Higher fat fruits and vegetables like avocado are fine in moderation.
- Beans and legumes – black beans, chickpeas, lentils
- Whole grains – whole grain bread and pasta, barley, brown rice, oats, quinoa

Chronic pancreatitis can often cause malnutrition as the pancreas doesn't function as effectively. You should be aware that Vitamins A, D, E, and K are most commonly found to be lacking due to pancreatitis. Vitamin deficiency due to malabsorption can cause osteoporosis, digestive problems and other symptoms.

Foods to Avoid

These are the sorts of foods you should limit or avoid:

- Organ meats – liver, kidneys, heart
- Fried foods – french fries, donuts and fried meats are high in saturated fats
- Processed meats – sausages and bacon
- Drinks with added sugar – fruit juices and soda
- Alcohol – alcohol consumption can worsen a pancreatitis attack acute and contribute to chronic pancreatitis
- Full-fat dairy – high-fat cheese (e.g cheddar and brie) and whole milk contains a lot of saturated fat
- High-fat spreads – margarine and butter

In particular, cooked or deep-fried foods may cause a pancreatitis flare-up. Refined grains such as white bread, flour and rice can also be problematic as they cause your insulin levels to spike.

Alcohol can also worsen an acute pancreatitis attack and contribute to chronic pancreatitis. Many of us drink too much already and heavy alcohol intake has been assocoiated with increased pancreatic cancer risk (1, 2, 3).

Choosing a Pancreatitis Diet

Some research says that some people can tolerate roughly 30-40% of their calories from fat when it's from whole-food plant sources or medium-chain triglycerides (MCT). Others may find they work better with less fat in their diet, but generally, you'll want a medium fat diet that's predominantly plant-based and low in saturated fats.

The Mediterranean diet fits this specification well. It focuses on the foods mentioned above and prioritises fats from healthy sources like extra virgin olive oil rather than saturated fats. Many leading organisations support eating a Mediterranean diet for pancreatitis as well as overall health, including:

- Harvard Medical School
- Cleveland Clinic
- Arthritis Foundation

- Mayo Clinic

It also consistently tops the best diets to follow, both because of how healthy it is and how sustainable it is to follow over the long-term. US News ranked it as the number 1 diet. This is great for people who want a long-term solution that they can stick to forever rather than a short-term fix. Various studies have shown that the Mediterranean diet can help with a range of health-related diseases, such as:

- Reduced risk of cardiovascular events,
- Reduced risk of coronary heart disease
- Reduced risk of developing type 2 diabetes
- Risk of breast cancer
- Reduced obesity
- Better cognitive function

Sample Menu

	Breakfast	Lunch	Dinner
Monday	Banana Yogurt Pots	Cannellini Bean Salad	Quick Moussaka
Tuesday	Tomato and Watermelon Salad	Edgy Veggie Wraps	Spicy Tomato Baked Eggs
Wednesday	Blueberry Oats Bowl Carrot	Orange and Avocado Salad	Salmon with Potatoes and Corn Salad
Thursday	Banana Yogurt Pots	Mixed Bean Salad	Spiced Carrot and Lentil Soup
Friday	Tomato and Watermelon Salad	Panzanella Salad Med Chicken	Quinoa and Greek Salad
Saturday	Blueberry Oats Bowl	Quinoa and Stir	Grilled Vegetables

		Fried Veg	with Bean Mash
Sunday	Banana Yogurt Pots	Moroccan Chickpea Soup	Spicy Mediterranean Beet Salad

Snacks are recommended between meal times. Some good snacks include:

- A handful of nuts or seeds
- A piece of fruit
- Carrots or baby carrots
- Berries or grapes

RECIPES

BANANA YOGURT POTS

Nutrition

- Calories – 236
- Protein – 14g
- Carbs – 32g
- Fat – 7g

Servings: 2

Prep time: 5 minutes

Ingredients

- 225g / ⅞ cup Greek yogurt
- 2 bananas, sliced into chunks
- 15g / 2 tbsp walnuts, toasted and chopped

Instructions

1. Place some of the yogurt into the bottom of a glass.
2. Add a layer of banana, then yogurt and repeat. Once the glass is full, scatter with the nuts.

CANNELLINI BEAN SALAD

Nutrition

- Calories – 302
- Protein – 20g
- Carbs – 54g
- Fat – 0g

Prep time: 5 minutes

Servings: 2

Ingredients

- 600g / 3 cups cannellini beans
- 70g / ⅜ cup cherry tomatoes, halved
- ½ red onion, thinly sliced
- ½ tbsp red wine vinegar
- small bunch basil, torn

Instructions

1. Rinse and drain the beans and mix with the tomatoes, onion and vinegar.
2. Season, then add basil just before serving.

MOUSSAKA

Nutrition

- Calories – 577
- Protein – 27g
- Carbs – 46g
- Fat – 27g

Prep time + cook time: 30 minutes

Servings: 2

Ingredients

- 1 tbsp extra virgin olive oil
- ½ onion, finely chopped
- 1 garlic clove, finely chopped
- 250g / 9 oz lean beef mince
- 200g can / 1 cup chopped tomatoes
- 1 tbsp tomato purée
- 1 tsp ground cinnamon
- 200g can / 1 cup chickpeas
- 100g pack / ⅔ cup feta cheese, crumbled
- Mint (fresh preferable)
- Brown bread, to serve

Instructions

1. Heat the oil in a pan. Add the onion and garlic and fry until soft. Add the mince and fry for 3-4 minutes until browned.
2. Tip the tomatoes into the pan and stir in the tomato purée and cinnamon, then season. Leave the mince to simmer for 20 minutes. Add the chickpeas halfway through.
3. Sprinkle the feta and mint over the mince. Serve with toasted bread.

TOMATO AND WATERMELON SALAD

Nutrition

- Calories – 177
- Protein – 5g
- Carbs – 13g
- Fat – 13g

Prep time + cook time: 5 minutes

Servings: 2

Ingredients

- 1 tbsp olive oil
- 1 tbsp red wine vinegar
- ¼ tsp chilli flakes
- 1 tbsp chopped mint
- 120g / ⅝ cup tomatoes, chopped
- ½ watermelon, cut into chunks
- 50g / ⅔ cup feta cheese, crumbled

Instructions

1. For the dressing, Mix the oil, vinegar, chilli flakes and mint and then season.
2. Put the tomatoes and watermelon into a bowl. Pour over the dressing, add the feta, then serve.

EDGY VEGGIE WRAPS

Nutrition

- Calories – 310
- Protein – 11g
- Carbs – 39g
- Fat – 11g

Prep time + cook time: 10 minutes

Servings: 2

Ingredients

- 100g / ½ cup cherry tomatoes
- 1 cucumber
- 6 Kalamata olives
- 2 large wholemeal tortilla wraps
- 50g / ¼ cup feta cheese
- 2 tbsp hummus

Instructions

1. Chop the tomatoes, cut the cucumber into sticks, split the olives and remove the stones.
2. Heat the tortillas.
3. Spread the houmous over the wrap. Put the vegetable mix in the middle and roll up.

SPICY TOMATO BAKED EGGS

Nutrition

- Calories – 417
- Protein – 19g
- Carbs – 45g
- Fat – 17g

Prep time + cook time: 25 minutes

Servings: 2

Ingredients

- 1 tbsp olive oil
- 2 red onions, chopped
- 1 red chilli, deseeded & chopped
- 1 garlic clove, sliced
- small bunch coriander, stalks and leaves chopped separately
- 800g can / 4 cups cherry tomatoes
- 4 eggs
- brown bread, to serve

Instructions

1. Heat the oil in a frying pan with a lid, then cook the onions, chilli, garlic and coriander stalks for 5 minutes until soft. Stir in the tomatoes, then simmer for 8-10 minutes.
2. Using the back of a large spoon, make 4 dips in the sauce, then crack an egg into each one. Put a lid on the pan, then cook over a low heat for 6-8 mins, until the eggs are done to your liking. Scatter with the coriander leaves and serve with bread.

BLUEBERRY OATS BOWL

Nutrition

- Calories – 235
- Protein – 13g
- Carbs – 38g
- Fat – 4g

Prep time + cook time: 10 minutes

Servings: 2

Ingredients

- 60g / ⅔ cup porridge oats
- 160g / ⅗ cup Greek yogurt
- 175g / ¾ blueberries
- 1 tsp honey

Instructions

1. Put the oats in a pan with 400ml of water. Heat and stir for about 2 minutes. Remove from the heat and add a third of the yogurt.
2. Tip the blueberries into a pan with the honey and 1 tbsp of water. Gently poach until the blueberries are tender.

3. Spoon the porridge into bowls and add the remaining yogurt and blueberries.

CARROT, ORANGE AND AVOCADO SALAD

Nutrition

- Calories – 177
- Protein – 5g
- Carbs – 13g
- Fat – 13g

Prep time + cook time: 5 minutes

Servings: 2

Ingredients

- 1 orange, plus zest and juice of 1
- 2 carrots, halved lengthways and sliced with a peeler
- 35g / 1 ½ cups rocket / arugula
- 1 avocado, stoned, peeled and sliced
- 1 tbsp olive oil

Instructions

1. Cut the segments from 1 of the oranges and put in a bowl with the carrots, rocket/arugula and avocado. Whisk together the orange juice,

zest and oil. Toss through the salad, and season

SALMON WITH POTATOES AND CORN SALAD

Nutrition

- Calories – 479
- Protein – 43g
- Carbs – 27g
- Fat – 21g

Prep time + cook time: 30 minutes

Servings: 2

Ingredients

- 200g / 1 ⅓ cups baby new potatoes
- 1 sweetcorn cob
- 2 skinless salmon fillets
- 60g / ⅓ cup tomatoes

- 1 tbsp red wine vinegar
- 1 tbsp extra-virgin olive oil
- Bunch of spring onions/scallions, finely chopped
- 1 tbsp capers, finely chopped
- handful basil leaves

Instructions

1. Cook potatoes in boiling water until tender, adding corn for final 5 minutes. Drain & cool.
2. For the dressing, mix the vinegar, oil, shallot, capers, basil & seasoning.
3. Heat grill to high. Rub some dressing on salmon & cook, skinned side down, for 7-8 minutes. Slice tomatoes & place on a plate. Slice the potatoes, cut the corn from the cob & add to plate. Add the salmon & drizzle over the remaining dressing.

MIXED BEAN SALAD

Nutrition

Calories – 240

Protein – 11g

Carbs – 22g

Fat – 12g

Prep time + cook time: 10 minutes

Servings: 2

Ingredients

- 145g / ⅘ cup jar artichoke heart in oil
- ½ tbsp sundried tomato paste
- ½ tsp red wine vinegar
- 200g can / 1 cup cannellini beans, drained and rinsed
- 150g / ¾ cup tomatoes, quartered
- handful Kalamata black olives
- 2 spring onions, thinly sliced on the diagonal
- 100g / ⅔ cup feta cheese, crumbled

Instructions

1. Drain the jar of artichokes, reserving 1-2 tbsp of oil. Add the oil, sun-dried tomato paste and vinegar and stir until smooth. Season to taste.
2. Chop the artichokes and tip into a bowl. Add the cannellini beans, tomatoes, olives, spring onions and half of the feta cheese. Stir in the artichoke oil mixture and tip into a serving bowl. Crumble over the remaining feta cheese, then serve.

SPICED CARROT AND LENTIL SOUP

Nutrition

- Calories – 238
- Protein – 11g
- Carbs – 34g
- Fat – 7g

Prep time + cook time: 25 minutes

Servings: 2

Ingredients

- 1 tsp cumin seeds
- pinch chilli flakes
- 1 tbsp olive oil
- 300g /2 cups carrots, washed and coarsely grated
- 70g / ⅓ cup split red lentils
- 500ml / 2 ¼ cups hot vegetable stock
- 60ml / ¼ cup milk
- Greek yogurt, to serve

Instructions

1. Heat a large saucepan and dry fry the cumin seeds and chilli flakes for 1 minute. Scoop out about half of the seeds with a spoon and set aside. Add the oil, carrot, lentils, stock and milk to the pan and bring to the boil. Simmer for 15 minutes until the lentils have swollen and softened.
2. Whizz the soup with a stick blender or in a food processor until smooth. Season to taste and finish with a dollop of Greek yogurt and a sprinkling of the reserved toasted spices.

PANZANELLE SALAD

Nutrition

- Calories – 452
- Protein – 6g
- Carbs – 37g
- Fat – 25g

Prep time + cook time: 10 minutes

Servings: 2

Ingredients

- 400g / 2 cups tomatoes
- 1 garlic clove, crushed
- 1 tbsp capers, drained and rinsed
- 1 ripe avocado, stoned, peeled and chopped
- 1 small red onion, very thinly sliced
- 2 slices of brown bread
- 2 tbsp olive oil
- 1 tbsp red wine vinegar
- small handful basil leaves

Instructions

1. Chop the tomatoes and put them in a bowl. Season well and add the garlic, capers, avocado and onion. Mix well and set aside for 10 minutes.
2. Meanwhile, tear the bread into chunks and place in a bowl. Drizzle over half of the olive oil and half of the vinegar. When ready to serve, scatter tomatoes and basil leaves and drizzle with remaining oil and vinegar. Stir before serving.

MED CHICKEN, QUINOA AND GREEK SALAD

Nutrition

- Calories – 473
- Protein – 36g
- Carbs – 57g
- Fat – 25g

Prep time + cook time: 20 minutes

Servings: 2

Ingredients

- 100g / ⅗ cup quinoa
- ½ red chilli, deseeded and finely chopped
- 1 garlic clove, crushed
- 2 chicken breasts
- 1 tbsp extra-virgin olive oil
- 150g / ¾ cup tomatoes, roughly chopped
- handful pitted black kalamata olives
- ½ red onion, finely sliced
- 50g / ½ cup feta cheese, crumbled
- small bunch mint leaves, chopped

- juice and zest ½ lemon

Instructions

1. Cook the quinoa following the pack instructions, then rinse in cold water and drain thoroughly.
2. Meanwhile, toss the chicken fillets in the olive oil with some seasoning, chilli and garlic. Lay in a hot pan and cook for 3-4 minutes each side or until cooked through. Transfer to a plate and set aside
3. Next, tip the tomatoes, olives, onion, feta and mint into a bowl. Toss in the cooked quinoa. Stir through the remaining olive oil, lemon juice and zest, and season well. Serve with the chicken on top.

QUINOA AND STIR FRIED VEG

Nutrition

- Calories – 473
- Protein – 11g
- Carbs – 56g
- Fat – 25g

Prep time + cook time: 30 minutes

Servings: 2

Ingredients

- 100g / ⅗ cup quinoa
- 3 tbsp olive oil
- 1 garlic clove, finely chopped
- 2 carrots, cut into thin sticks
- 150g / 1 ⅔ leek, sliced
- 1 broccoli head, cut into small florets
- 50g / ¼ cup tomatoes
- 100ml / ¼ cup vegetable stock
- 1 tsp tomato purée
- juice ½ lemon

Instructions

1. Cook the quinoa according to pack instructions. Meanwhile, heat 3 tbsp of the oil in a pan, then add the garlic and quickly fry for 1 minute. Throw in the carrots, leeks and broccoli, then stir-fry for 2 minutes until everything is glistening.
2. Add the tomatoes, mix together the stock and tomato purée, then add to the pan. Cover and cook for 3 minutes. Drain the quinoa and toss in the remaining oil and lemon juice. Divide between warm plates and spoon the vegetables on top.

GRILLED VEGETABLE WITH BEAN MASH

Nutrition

- Calories – 314
- Protein – 19g
- Carbs – 33g
- Fat – 16g

Prep time + cook time: 40 minutes

Servings: 2

Ingredients

- 1 pepper, deseeded & quartered
- 1 aubergine, sliced lengthways
- 2 courgettes, sliced lengthways
- 2 tbsp olive oil
- For the mash
- 400g / 2 cups haricot beans, rinsed
- 1 garlic clove, crushed
- 100ml / ½ cup vegetable stock
- 1 tbsp chopped coriander

Instructions

1. Heat the grill. Arrange the vegetables over a grill pan &brush lightly with oil. Grill until lightly browned, turn them over, brush again with oil, then grill until tender.
2. Meanwhile, put the beans in a pan with garlic and stock. Bring to the boil, then simmer, uncovered, for 10 minutes. Mash roughly with a potato masher. Divide the vegetables and mash between 2 plates, drizzle over oil and sprinkle with black pepper and coriander.

MOROCCAN CHICKPEA SOUP

Nutrition

- Calories – 408
- Protein – 15g
- Carbs – 63g
- Fat – 11g

Prep time + cook time: 25 minutes

Servings: 2

Ingredients

- 1 tbsp olive oil
- ½ medium onion, chopped
- 1 celery sticks, chopped
- 1 tsp ground cumin
- 300ml / 1 ¼ cups hot vegetable stock
- 200g can / 1 cup chopped tomatoes
- 200g can / 1 cup chickpeas, rinsed and drained
- 50g / ¼ cup frozen broad beans
- zest and juice ½ lemon
- coriander & bread to serve

Instructions

1. Heat the oil in a saucepan, then fry the onion and celery for 10 minutes until softened. Add the cumin and fry for another minute.
2. Turn up the heat, then add the stock, tomatoes, chickpeas and black pepper. Simmer for 8 minutes. Add broad beans and lemon juice and cook for a further 2 minutes. Top with lemon zest and coriander.

SPICY MEDITERRANEAN BEET SALAD

Nutrition

- Calories – 548
- Protein – 23g
- Carbs – 58g
- Fat – 20g

Prep time + cook time: 40 minutes

Servings: 2

Ingredients

- 8 raw baby beetroots, or 4 medium, scrubbed
- ½ tbsp sumac
- ½ tbsp ground cumin
- 400g can / 2 cups chickpeas, drained and rinsed
- 2 tbsp olive oil
- ½ tsp lemon zest
- ½ tsp lemon juice
- 200g / ½ cup Greek yogurt
- 1 tbsp harissa paste
- 1 tsp crushed red chilli flakes
- mint leaves, chopped, to serve

Instructions

1. Heat oven to 220C/200C fan/ gas 7. Halve or quarter beetroots depending on size. Mix spices together. On a large baking tray, mix chickpeas and beetroot with the oil. Season with salt & sprinkle over the spices. Mix again. Roast for 30 minutes.
2. While the vegetables are cooking, mix the lemon zest and juice with the yogurt. Swirl the harissa through and spread into a bowl. Top with the beetroot & chickpeas, and sprinkle with the chilli flakes & mint.

APPLE BUTTERNUT SQUASH PANCAKES

These delicious pancakes can be used as a meal any time of the day. They are rich in beta-carotene and are designed to be easy to tolerate for pancreatic cancer symptoms such as nausea and overall stomach upset. For additional protein, nuts can be added. For those who are experiencing fat intolerance, reduced fat versions of the dairy components can be substituted, along with lower lactose alternatives for those with lactose intolerance.

For those on more severe fiber restrictions, the apple and squash components can also be peeled and boiled to help break down some of the fibers for optimal digestive tolerance. These can also be easily frozen (with layers of parchment paper in between) and reheated in the toaster oven or microwave.

Yield: 12 small pancakes (6 large)

Ingredients

- 3 cups grated raw butternut squash or acorn squash (may also use zucchini)
- 1 large green apple (or 2 small) grated, raw

- 1/3 cup sour cream (use reduced-fat or vegan sour cream if necessary)
- egg
- 1/4 cup milk of choice (use lactose-free, non-dairy, or reduced-fat as needed)
- 1 cup all-purpose flour 1 tsp. baking powder
- 1 tsp. baking soda
- 1 tsp. cinnamon

INSTRUCTIONS

1. Grate squash on cheese grater or food processor. Steam in a shallow bowl in microwave with a small amount of water for 3 minutes to soften.
2. Core and grate apple on cheese grater or food processor, and add to squash mixture.
3. Add squash and apple to a mixing bowl and stir in sour cream, egg, and milk with a fork.
4. In a separate bowl, sift flour, baking powder, baking soda, and cinnamon. Add to mixing bowl and stir with the fork.
5. Heat frying pan to low-medium and spray with cooking spray.

6. Using a ladle or a spoon, drop batter onto pan into small pancakes. Flip when bubbles start to form around the edges of pancake.

NUTRITION

- calories 166
- fat 3.9 grams
- saturated fat 2.1 grams
- cholesterol 34 mg,
- carbohydrate 29.8 grams
- dietary fiber 2.9 grams
- protein 4.4 grams

PASTIERA (PASTA EGG BAKE)

Pastiera is traditionally an Italian-style Easter cake that is sweetened and made with ricotta cheese. This recipe is a savory spin on this classic dish and is packed with protein from the eggs and milk. Lactose-free milk and cheese can be used for those experiencing lactose intolerance. Spaghetti squash is also a great substitution for pasta noodles as a lower carbohydrate alternative or for those looking to add a tolerable vegetable component.

Yield: 8 servings

Ingredients

- 12 eggs, beaten (may substitute for lower fat pasteurized liquid egg product)
- 2 cups of milk (substitute non-fat or reduced fat milk if experiencing fat intolerance)
- Salt and pepper to taste
- 1 cup of grated Parmesan cheese
- Perciatelli (aka Bucatini or #6 macaroni spaghetti with a hole running through)

INSTRUCTIONS

1. Preheat oven to 250°. Spray a rectangular 9x13" baking dish with nonfat cooking spray.
2. Cook pasta according to package directions.
3. Mix beaten eggs with milk, salt, pepper, and cheese while macaroni is cooking.
4. Combine together in the 9x13" baking dish.
5. Bake at 250° for 10 minutes, and then increase oven temperature to 350° for 25-30 minutes.
6. Cut into 8 pieces, or smaller as a side dish.

NUTRITION

- calories 378
- fat 11.5 grams
- saturated fat 4.6 grams
- cholesterol 259 mg
- carbohydrate 48.5 grams
- dietary fiber 2 grams
- protein 21.4 grams

THANKSGIVING MEATBALLS

This is a unique twist to a comfort food that takes meatballs from savory to slightly sweet. It's a great choice for those needing low-fat protein choices during the holiday.

Yield: 16 medium sized meatballs, 8 servings

INGREDIENTS

- 1 1/2 lb. ground turkey meat (you can use half ground turkey and half sweet turkey sausage for extra flavor)
- 1 1/4 cup of herbed stuffing bread
- cubes
- 1/2 cup dried cranberries
- 1 large egg plus 1 egg white
- 1/4 cup finely chopped sweet onion
- 1 Tbsp. chopped fresh sage
- 1 tsp. salt
- 1 Tbsp. olive oil
- Other add-in ideas: shredded carrots or chopped mushrooms

INSTRUCTIONS

1. Preheat oven to 450°.
2. Coat a 9x13 inch baking sheet with olive oil
1. and set aside.
2. In a large bowl, combine the ground turkey/turkey sausage, cranberries, eggs, onion, sage, and salt. Add half of the stuffing cubes in whole form, and crush the other half in your hands to resemble bread crumbs. Mix everything together with your hands until it is all incorporated.
3. Coat your hands with a little bit of olive oil and roll the mixture firmly into balls about the size of golf balls. Place the meatballs in the baking dish directly next to each other in rows. This will help them keep their shape while baking.
4. Roast for about 20 minutes, until the meatballs are cooked through and slightly brown on top.
5. Serve meatballs with gravy and cranberry sauce, and enjoy!

NUTRITION

- calories 192
- fat 7.9 grams
- saturated fat 1.8 grams
- cholesterol 73 mg,
- carbohydrate 5.4 grams
- dietary fiber 0.9 grams
- protein 18.5 grams

MAPLE GREEN BEANS

Roasting green beans is a quick and easy way to prepare a delicious green vegetable. This recipe can be made with fresh out-of-the-garden green beans, fresh packaged and pre-washed green beans, or frozen green beans. Boost the flavor by using pure maple syrup.

Yield: 4 Servings

NUTRITION

- calories 59
- fat 1.3 grams
- saturated fat 0 grams
- cholesterol 0 mg,
- carbohydrate 11.5 grams
- dietary fiber 3.9 grams
- protein 2.1 grams

INGREDIENTS

- 1 lb. green beans
- 1 Tbsp. maple syrup

- 1 tsp. olive oil
- 1/2 tsp. salt
- 1/4 tsp. pepper

INSTRUCTIONS

1. Preheat oven to 400°.
2. In a large bowl, toss green beans with maple
1. syrup, oil, salt and pepper.
2. Arrange evenly on sheet tray.
3. Roast until tender, about 20 to 25 minutes.

CARROT PURÉE WITH OLIVE OIL AND CILANTRO

This is the perfect side dish for the holiday season, especially for patients facing pancreatic cancer, as it is a well-cooked vegetable dish which is easier to digest and less likely to aggravate digestive issues. The carrots provide an excellent source of beta-carotene. The oil may be reduced if sensitive to fat, or coconut oil may be substituted (which may be more easily absorbed). If you are sensitive to additional herbed flavors, the cilantro can be reduced or omitted. This purée can also translate well to any other root vegetable or squash – such as turnip, parsnip, acorn squash, or butternut squash. Yield: 6 servings

NUTRITION

- calories 142
- fat 11.7 grams
- saturated fat 1.7 grams
- cholesterol 0 mg
- carbohydrate 10 grams,
- dietary fiber 2.5 grams, protein 0.8 grams

INGREDIENTS

- About 10 carrots, peeled and cubed
- 5 Tbsp. extra virgin olive oil
- Sea salt
- Fresh black pepper
- 3 Tbsp. finely chopped fresh cilantro
- (may substitute other fresh herbs of choice and as tolerated)

INSTRUCTIONS

1. In a large pot, boil peeled and cubed carrots for about 20 minutes until they are very tender. (Alternatively, steaming them in a steam pan over boiling water may preserve the maximum amount of nutrients.)
2. In a medium pan, add fresh cilantro leaves and 3 Tbsp. of extra virgin olive oil. Heat on lowest flame for about 5 minutes.
3. Remove from heat and allow to sit for about 5 minutes. Remove cilantro from oil and set aside.
4. In a food processor or using an immersion blender, add in cooked carrots and cilantro

10. oil and 2 Tbsp. of extra virgin olive oil. Purée
11. until smooth.
5. Add sea salt and fresh black pepper to taste
12. and fresh cilantro as a garnish.

HEARTY VEGETABLE AND LENTIL SOUP

This hearty soup is very versatile and can be adapted for whatever vegetables you have available. Use this dish as a complement to a meal or serve with homemade corn bread to complete a meal. The vegetables and lentils provide an excellent amount of insoluble and soluble fiber, and this dish is a great choice for those dealing with constipation.

Yield: 6 servings

INGREDIENTS

- 3 cups water
- 3 cups vegetable or chicken broth
- 3 medium carrots, chopped
- 1 medium onion, chopped
- 1 cup dried lentils, rinsed
- 2 celery ribs, sliced
- 1 small bell pepper, color of your choice
- 1/4 cup uncooked brown rice
- 1 tsp. dried basil or 1 Tbsp. of fresh
- chopped basil
- 1 garlic clove, minced

- 1 bay leaf
- 1/2 cup tomato paste

INSTRUCTIONS

1. In a large saucepan, combine all ingredients except tomato paste. Bring to a boil.
2. Reduce heat; cover and simmer for 1 to 1 1/2 hours or until lentils and rice are tender.
3. Add the tomato paste and stir until blended.
4. Cook for 10-15 minutes. Discard bay leaf.

NUTRITION

- calories 206
- fat 1.4 grams
- saturated fat 0 grams
- cholesterol 0 mg
- carbohydrate 36 grams
- dietary fiber 12.6 grams
- protein 12.9 grams

TURKEY MEATLOAF (MINI)

This healthy alternative to beef meatloaf is adaptable to those dealing with a variety of treatment-related symptoms. Providing a generous amount of protein and flavored with vegetables, this meatloaf is sure to satisfy. This is a good selection for those dealing with gastrointestinal upset like nausea or diarrhea and for those needing blander flavors and less aroma. If you are looking to spice it up, consider adding red pepper flakes, hot sauce, or your favorite BBQ sauce. If looking for a lower-fat alternative, you can use turkey breast meat and add 1/4 cup more broth to this recipe for moistness.

Yield: 8 servings

INGREDIENTS

- 1 Tbsp. olive oil
- 2 lb. ground turkey (for a leaner preference use 1 lb. breast and 1 lb. dark meat or 2 lb. breast meat for most lean option)
- 1 large or 2 small zucchini
- 2 carrots

- 1/2 medium onion
- 1 cup quick cook oats
- 3/4 cup turkey or chicken broth
- 1 Tbsp. Worcestershire sauce
- 1 Tbsp. ketchup
- 1 egg
- 1 tsp. salt
- 1 tsp. pepper

INSTRUCTIONS

1. Preheat oven to 375°.
2. Shred zucchini and carrot. Slice onion finely. Alternatively, you can chop ingredients in a mini food processor.
3. Sauté vegetables in olive oil on medium heat until softened, approximately 3 to 4 minutes.
4. While vegetables cook, add broth to oats and let soak.
5. Add cooked vegetables, oats, ketchup, Worcestershire sauce, egg, salt, and pepper to ground turkey.
6. Mix ingredients together, avoid overmixing.

7. Place mixture in a meatloaf shape in a rectangular baking dish and bake for 1 hour and internal thermometer reads at least 165°. For extra crispy top, broil for the last 5 minutes of cooking, watching closely to avoid burning.

TIP: you can also make "mini meatloafs" in a muffin pan or miniature loaf pans, or even on a sheet pan shaped into 8 smaller loafs. These are great for freezing and lend themselves well to a leftover meatloaf sandwich.

NUTRITION

- calories 324
- fat 16.3 grams
- saturated fat 2.8 grams
- cholesterol 146 mg
- carbohydrate 11.6 grams
- dietary fiber 2 grams
- protein 37.8 grams

SWEET POTATO AND WHITE BEAN FRITTERS

Trying this unique plant-based recipe will add vibrancy and texture to your plate. Substitute any squash or beans that you have available. This recipe is a good choice for those needing foods that are soft and easy to chew and swallow.

Yield: 12 fritters

INGREDIENTS

- 2 cups (10 oz.) cubed and peeled sweet potato
- 1 can (15.5 oz.) no-added salt white beans, drained and rinsed
- 4 Tbsp. quick cooking oats
- 1 large egg
- 1/4 cup onion, minced
- 1 large clove garlic, minced
- 2 tsp. chopped fresh sage leaves
- 1/4 tsp. cumin Salt and freshly ground pepper to taste
- 1 Tbsp. canola oil or extra virgin olive oil, divided

- 3/4 cup low-fat sour cream or fat-free plain Greek-style yogurt

INSTRUCTIONS

1. In large saucepan with a steamer basket, steam sweet potatoes until tender, about 15-17 minutes.
2. Transfer sweet potato to food processor. Add beans, oats, egg, onion, garlic, sage, cumin. Pulse until blended yet slightly chunky.
3. Season with salt and pepper.
4. Heat 1 Tbsp. oil in large skillet over medium-high heat.
5. Gently drop six 1/4 cup portions of mixture into pan and gently press into round patties with back of measuring cup or spatula. Don't over crowd skillet.
6. Sauté fritters until golden brown on bottom, about 5 minutes. Heat may need to be adjusted for optimal browning.
7. Carefully turn over each fritter and sauté until other side is golden brown, about 3-4 minutes.

8. Transfer fritters to plate and cover with foil to keep warm.
9. Use remaining oil to sauté remaining six fritters. There should be 12 fritters in total. Serve warm with sour cream or Greek yogurt.

NUTRITION

- calories 104
- fat 4.9 grams,
- saturated fat 2.1 grams
- cholesterol 22 mg
- carbohydrate 12.5 grams
- dietary fiber 2.7 grams
- protein 3.7 grams

RICE PUDDING

A creamy, often well-tolerated, high-calorie pudding that works as a great dessert for those needing to add protein and calories to their daily intake. For those requiring a lower fat alternative, reduced-fat milk may be substituted. Non-dairy, lactose-free options like soy, rice, or almond milk can work as well.

Yield: 4 servings

INGREDIENTS

- 2 cups of whole milk, reduced-fat milk, or non-dairy alternative
- 1/3 cup of sugar
- 3/4 cups of long grain white or brown rice
- 1/4 tsp. salt
- 1 egg (beaten)
- 1/2 tsp. vanilla extract
- 1/4 cup dried fruit of your choice (optional)
- Cinnamon or nutmeg for sprinkling on top (optional)

Tip: for extra cinnamon flavor, boil rice with a cinnamon stick added to the water

INSTRUCTIONS

1. First rinse uncooked rice with cold water.
2. Bring 1 1/2 cups of water to a boil.
3. Add rice, reduce heat, and cook for approximately 20 minutes until tender.
4. In large pot add rice, 1 1/2 cups milk, sugar and salt.
5. Stir rice constantly to avoid rice from sticking to bottom of pot.
6. Cook until mixture is a thick and creamy texture, approximately 20 minutes.
7. Remove pot from heat, and while still hot, add remaining 1/2 cup milk, beaten eggs (add very slowly while stirring pot), vanilla, and optional dried fruit (such as raisins).
8. Return to medium heat and stir again until slightly thickened (5-10 minutes max).
9. Remove from heat, and pour into containers. Top with a sprinkling of cinnamon or nutmeg for garnish as desired.

10. Refrigerate before serving.

NUTRITION

- calories 289
- fat 5.9 grams
- saturated fat 0.5 grams
- cholesterol 59 mg
- carbohydrate 50 grams,
- dietary fiber 1.2 grams
- protein 8.1 grams

BANANA BLUEBERRY MUFFINS

These muffins are a great quick breakfast treat, with bananas and blueberries providing soluble fiber, potassium, and phytonutrients. Non-dairy milk can be substituted for those who are intolerant to lactose and whole-wheat flour can be substituted to increase the fiber content.

Yield: 12 muffins

INGREDIENTS

- 1/2 cup mashed ripe banana (about 1 large)
- 1/2 cup granulated sugar
- 1/2 cup milk (may also sub any non-dairy milk)
- 1/3 cup canola oil
- 1 Tbsp. vanilla extract
- 1 tsp. cinnamon
- 1 cup all-purpose flour (or whole wheat flour)
- 2 tsp. baking powder
- 1/2 cup frozen blueberries

INSTRUCTIONS

1. Preheat oven to 400°.
2. Line muffin pan with paper cups.
3. In a large bowl, mash the banana with a fork.
4. Add the sugar, milk, oil, vanilla, cinnamon, and whisk until combined.
5. Add the flour, baking powder, and stir until just combined; don't over mix.
6. Fold in 1/2 cup frozen blueberries.
7. Add batter to muffin tin (for easy distribution use medium cookie scoop)
8. Bake for 15-20 minutes, or until tops are slightly golden.

NUTRITION

- calories 125
- fat 6.4 grams
- saturated fat 0.6 grams
- cholesterol 1 mg
- carbohydrate 15.5 grams
- dietary fiber 0.7 grams
- protein 1.5 grams

BAKED BERRY FRENCH TOAST

This French toast recipe is great to make ahead of time for a busy weekday morning. It is a good balanced entrée that includes protein, carbohydrates, dairy, and fruit. Cream cheese and milk components can be substituted with lactose-free versions for those experiencing lactose intolerance.

Yield: 8 Servings

INGREDIENTS

- 12 slices day-old bread, cut into 1-inch cubes
- 1 (12 oz.) package of low-fat cream cheese, room temperature
- 2 1/4 cups low-fat fat-free milk or non-dairy alternative, divided
- 2 tsp. vanilla, divided
- 2 cups blueberries, fresh or thawed frozen, divided
- 10 eggs, beaten
- 1/4 cup plus 1 Tbsp. honey or pure maple syrup

INSTRUCTIONS

1. Preheat oven to 350°.
2. Lightly grease a 9x13 inch-baking dish.
3. Blend 1 brick of cream cheese, 1/4 cup of milk, 1 Tbsp. honey and 1 tsp. vanilla.
4. Arrange 1/2 of the bread cubes in bottom of dish. Top with cream cheese mixture.
5. Sprinkle 1 cup of blueberries over top, and top with remaining bread cubes.
6. In large bowl, mix eggs, milk, vanilla extract, and honey or syrup. Pour over bread cubes Cover, refrigerate 1 hour or overnight.
7. Cover, and bake for 30 minutes. Uncover, and continue baking for 25-30 minutes, until center is firm and surface is lightly browned.
8. Let cool for 10-12 minutes. Top with remaining berries and enjoy.

NUTRITION

- calories 231
- fat 7.5 grams
- saturated fat 1.7 grams
- cholesterol 205 mg

- carbohydrate 29 grams
- dietary fiber 3.8 grams
- protein 13.7 grams

PUMPKIN OATMEAL BARS

These are a healthy alternative to many common cookie recipes. Whole-wheat flour, oats, pumpkin, and ground flaxseed add soluble and insoluble fiber, along with the phytochemical and antioxidant benefits of the added spices. Great selections for an after dinner dessert or midday snack. Flaxseed can be omitted if experiencing gas, bloating, or diarrhea.

Yield: 40 square bars or 48 cookies

INGREDIENTS

- 2 cups whole-wheat flour
- 1 1/3 cups rolled oats
- 1 tsp. baking soda
- 3/4 tsp. salt

- 1 tsp. cinnamon
- 1/2 tsp. nutmeg
- 1 1/3 cup sugar
- 2/3 cup canola oil
- 3 Tbsp. molasses
- 1 can of cooked pumpkin puree
- 1 tsp. vanilla
- 2 Tbsp. ground flaxseed (optional)
- Optional add-ins: 1 cup mini chocolate chips

INSTRUCTIONS

1. Preheat oven to 350°. Grease two 12 x 17 baking sheet pans.
2. Mix together flour, oats, baking soda, salt, and spices.
3. In a separate bowl, mix together sugar, oil, molasses, pumpkin, vanilla, and optional flaxseeds until very well combined.
4. Mix flour and sugar mixtures together. Fold in chocolate chips, if desired.
5. Spread and press batter onto greased cookie sheets (to make cookies, drop 1 inch size balls of batter an inch apart, and flatten tops of

cookies with fork or your fingers to press into cookie shape).
6. Bake for 16 minutes or until inserted knife or toothpick is clean. Rotate halfway through baking.
7. Remove from oven (if making cookies, transfer to wire rack to cool).
8. Once cool slice into 20 bars per sheet pan.

NUTRITION

- calories 101
- fat 4 grams
- saturated fat 0 grams
- cholesterol 0 mg
- carbohydrate 15.4 grams
- dietary fiber 0.9 grams
- protein 1.2 grams

ASPARAGUS FRITTATA

Frittatas are very versatile – they can be used at any meal as a main dish, side dish or appetizer, and can easily be turned into a quiche by adding a pie crust at the bottom (if able to tolerate higher amounts of fat). Eggs provide the highest quality protein available in any food. This recipe is great for those needing easy to chew/swallowing foods.

Yield: 1 9-inch quiche, serves 6

INGREDIENTS

- 1/2 lb. fresh asparagus, trimmed and cut into 1/2 inch pieces
- 1 egg white, lightly beaten
- 4 eggs, beaten
- 1 1/2 cups fat-free or low-fat milk
- 1/4 tsp. ground nutmeg
- 1 Tbsp. Dijon mustard
- 1 cup shredded Swiss or muenster cheese (use reduced fat cheese if experiencing fat intolerance)
- Salt and pepper to taste

INSTRUCTIONS

1. Preheat oven to 375°.
2. Add asparagus to saucepan with 1 inch of water or place in a steamer. Steam for 4-6 minutes or until tender but not mushy. Once steamed, allow it to drain well and cool.
3. Coat pie dish with nonstick cooking spray.
4. Add drained and dried asparagus to pie dish.
5. In a bowl, beat together eggs, milk, mustard, nutmeg, salt and pepper. Add shredded cheese and mix in.
6. Pour egg mixture into pie pan.
7. Bake uncovered in preheated oven until firm, about 40-50 minutes.
8. Enjoy warm or at room temperature.

NUTRITION

- calories 125
- fat 8.8 grams
- saturated fat 4.6 grams
- cholesterol 127 mg,
- carbohydrate 2.2 grams
- dietary fiber 0.9 grams

- protein 9.9 grams

VEGETABLE POPOVER

These vegetable popovers are excellent for individuals needing soft, easy-to-swallow foods. Eggs (or egg substitute) add an excellent source of high-quality protein. This is also a great recipe to prepare ahead of time and reheat as a healthy mini-meal.

Yield: 6 servings

INGREDIENTS

- 1 zucchini, chopped into bite-size pieces
- 1 large carrot, chopped into small pieces (about half the size of the zucchini)
- 2 tsp. olive oil
- 6 large eggs
- 1/4 cup milk (non-dairy alternative, if desired)
- 1/3 cup shredded cheddar cheese (use reduced-fat cheese for those experiencing fat

intolerance) Salt and freshly ground black pepper, to taste
- Pinch of turmeric
- Onion powder, to taste

INSTRUCTIONS

1. Preheat the oven to 350°.
2. Spray 6 muffin cups with nonstick spray.
3. Sauté the zucchini and the carrots in 2 tsp. olive oil for 5-7 minutes.
4. In a medium bowl, whisk together the eggs and milk. Add salt, pepper, turmeric, and onion powder.
5. Distribute egg mixture evenly into muffin cups.
6. Distribute zucchini and carrots into egg mixture.
7. Bake 25 to 30 minutes, or until egg is cooked through.

NUTRITION

- calories 126
- fat 8.9 grams

- saturated fat 3.2 grams
- cholesterol 193 mg
- carbohydrate 3.4 grams
- dietary fiber 0.7 grams
- protein 8.7 grams

EDAMAME HUMMUS WRAP

Soy is a high-quality protein that does not cause the same discomfort that other beans and hummuses can. This recipe is extremely easy and satisfying. Can be delicious plain or with any added vegetables that you can tolerate (those with diarrhea or indigestion should be sure to use well-cooked vegetables without the skin).

Yield: 4 servings

INGREDIENTS

- 1 cup cooked shelled edamame
- 1/4 cup Tahini (sesame paste)

- 1 Tbsp. lemon juice Garlic clove, peeled
- 2 Tbsp. coarsely chopped fresh herbs (such as rosemary, thyme, and basil)
- 2 Tbsp. olive oil
- Salt to taste (approximately 1/4 tsp.)
- 4 flour wraps

Optional: Sautéed or roasted vegetables, or fresh, raw vegetables that you can tolerate

INSTRUCTIONS

1. Combine edamame, tahini, lemon juice, garlic, and herbs in food processor.
2. Process ingredients until smooth.
3. Drizzle olive oil through feed tube of food processor, continuing to process until the oil is fully incorporated into the hummus mixture.
4. Season with salt to taste.
5. Spread 1/4 cup hummus in each wrap, top with raw or roasted vegetables of choice, roll and serve.

NUTRITION

- calories 399

- fat 21.9 grams
- saturated fat 3.1 grams
- cholesterol 0 mg
- carbohydrate 39.9 grams
- dietary fiber 4.1 grams
- protein 12.1 grams

SALMON BURGER WITH BOK CHOY, GINGER AND LEMONGRASS

Salmon burgers provide a tasty alternative to old-fashioned beef burgers along with the benefit of healthy omega-3 fats. These burgers have a refreshing appeal from the lemongrass and ginger. Top with traditional plant-based burger toppings on a hearty whole-grain roll. Tuna can be substituted for salmon as well. For those sensitive to spices, they can be toned down as needed.

Yield: 4 Servings

INGREDIENTS

- 1 lb. salmon fillet (or canned salmon)
- 3 cups bok choy, chopped finely (green leafy top only)
- 3 scallions, minced
- 1 Tbsp. finely grated ginger (peeled)
- 1 Tbsp. finely grated lemongrass (dried lemongrass can be substituted if fresh is not found)
- Salt and pepper to taste

- 1 large egg white
- 1 Tbsp. soy sauce
- Cilantro (optional)

INSTRUCTIONS

1. Cut salmon into 1/4 inch dice (or use canned salmon), stir into mixture of bok choy, scallions, ginger, lemongrass, salt and pepper in large bowl until combined.
2. Beat together egg white and soy sauce in a small bowl and stir into salmon mixture.
3. Form into four patties that are 1/2 inch thick.
4. Heat non-stick skillet over medium heat. Add 1 Tbsp. of olive oil to cover bottom of skillet. Add salmon patties, cooking for approximately 3-4 minutes per side.
5. Serve hot.
6. Top with cilantro leaves, if desired.

NUTRITION

- calories 173
- fat 7.2 grams
- saturated fat 1 gram

- cholesterol 50 mg,
- carbohydrate 3.6 grams
- dietary fiber 1 gram
- protein 24.3 grams

PEACHES AND CREAM SMOOTHIE

Simple meals like shakes and smoothies are often helpful ways for people caring for or living with pancreatic cancer to get the nutrients they need. This Peaches and Cream Smoothie combines the potassium and fiber benefits of peaches and bananas along with soluble fiber from rolled oats, which can help to alleviate loose bowel movements and promote regularity. The protein powder can be added at the recommendation of your healthcare team for additional nutritional value. Dairy components can be easily substituted with lactose-free or non-dairy versions.

Yield: 1-2 servings

INGREDIENTS

- ½ cup rolled oats
- cup plain yogurt (or soy/coconut/almond yogurt)
- ¾ cup milk (or soy/almond/rice milk) + ¼ cup more for morning

- 1 small ripe peach (or ½ cup frozen peaches, thawed and softened)
- ½ medium banana
- Pinch of salt
- 1-2 Tbsp. protein powder (whey or soy) (optional)

INSTRUCTIONS

1. Gather all ingredients
2. Combine ingredients in a blender and enjoy
3. Store in a container in your refrigerator overnight if making ahead of time. In the morning, add last ¼ cup milk, more if you need it to blend smoothly.

Nutrition

(assumes regular whole milk and yogurt)

- calories 426
- fat 9 grams
- saturated fat 4.5 grams
- cholesterol 25 mg
- carbohydrate 68 grams
- dietary fiber 7 grams

- protein 20 grams

TURKEY SWEET POTATO HASH

Since fatigue is sometimes experienced by people living with pancreatic cancer, this easy-to-prepare dish is nutrient dense and a good source of protein and B vitamins, which can help boost energy. In addition, the cooked apple and sweet potato provide fiber that is easily tolerated and full of antioxidants like beta-carotene and quercetin. The ingredients include a variety of appealing textures and flavors of the holiday season!

Yield: 6 servings, 1 ¼ cups each

INGREDIENTS

- 2 medium sweet potatoes, peeled and cut into ½-inch pieces

- 1 medium apple, cored and cut into ½-inch pieces (Honeycrisp or Braeburn work wonderfully, although any apple can suit this recipe)
- ½ cup reduced-fat sour cream (may also substitute reduced-fat yogurt)
- 1 tsp. lemon juice
- 1 Tbsp. olive oil
- 1 medium shallot, chopped
- 3 cups diced, cooked, skinless turkey breast (or chicken)
- 1 tsp. dried rosemary (1 Tbsp. fresh, chopped)
- Salt and pepper, to taste

INSTRUCTIONS

1. Place sweet potatoes in a steamer basket and cook for approximately 10 minutes.
2. Add apple and cook until everything is just tender, about 3 minutes longer. Be sure that they are not overly mushy. Drain and set aside.
3. Transfer 1 cup of the mixture to a large bowl; mash. Stir in sour cream and lemon juice.

4. Add the remaining sweet potato/apple mixture and stir gently to mix.
5. Heat oil in a large skillet over medium-high heat. Add shallot until softened, 1 to 2 minutes.
6. Add turkey (or chicken), rosemary, salt and pepper.
7. Stir mixture occasionally and cook until heated through, about 2 minutes.
8. Add the reserved sweet potato apple mixture to the pan. Press on the hash with a wide metal spoon or spatula. Cook hash until the bottom is lightly browned, about 3 minutes.
9. Divide into multiple sections with spatula; flip and cook until the bottom sides are browned, about 2 to 3 minutes.
7. Serve promptly

Nutrition

- calories 174
- fat 6 grams
- saturated fat 2 grams
- cholesterol 38 mg

- carbohydrate 17 grams
- dietary fiber 2 grams,
- protein 14 grams.

TURKEY TORTELLINI SOUP

Many people with pancreatic cancer often will better tolerate and enjoy simple, comforting meals. This classic soup recipe can be the base for a warm and hearty soup.

Yield: 8 Servings

INGREDIENTS

- One 12-15 lb. turkey
- 3 medium-size onions
- 6 garlic cloves
- 6 large carrots
- 1 head of celery
- 3 bay leaves
- 6 sprigs fresh thyme

- 1 sprig rosemary
- 3 cups cheese tortellini
- 1 bunch parsley
- ½ cup parmigiano cheese
- ¼ cup extra virgin olive oil

INSTRUCTIONS

For Roasting the Turkey

1. Preheat oven to 350°.
2. Place turkey on roasting rack. Season inside and out with salt and pepper.
3. Roast turkey for 2 ½ or 3 hours until internal temperature reaches 155°, basting with natural juices every 30 minutes.
4. Remove turkey and lightly dome with aluminum foil. Allow to cool.
5. Once cool, remove skin and debone turkey.
6. Place body and all bones back into the roasting pan. Roast at 350° for 30 minutes, until bones are dark, golden brown.
7. Shred turkey meat into bite size pieces.
8. Reserve.

For the Turkey Stock

1. In a large stock pot, place turkey bones and body, ½ head of celery (chopped), 3 carrots (chopped), 2 onions (chopped), 4 garlic cloves (smashed), 3 bay leaves, 1 sprig rosemary and 6 sprigs thyme.
2. Cover with 4 inches of water, bring to a simmer.
3. Lower heat and slowly simmer stock for 2 hours, occasionally skimming fat from the top.
4. After 2 hours, strain stock through a fine sift and cheese cloth.
5. Cool and reserve.

For the Garnish

1. Remaining celery, small dice (quarter by quarter inch)
2. Remaining carrots, small dice (quarter by quarter inch)
3. Remaining onions, small dice (quarter by quarter inch)
4. Remaining garlic, minced

5. In a large stock pot, put 2 gallons of water. Add 2 Tbsp. of kosher salt. Bring to a rolling boil and add the tortellini.
6. Cook for 6 minutes, occasionally stirring. Strain.
7. Toss 1 Tbsp. extra virgin olive oil into the tortellini.
8. Lay flat on a sheet tray and allow to cool in refrigerator.
9. Reserve.

To Assemble the Soup

1. Add stock to large stock pot.
2. Add all diced vegetables and bring to a simmer. Cook until carrots are tender, approximately 6-8 minutes.

3. Add shredded turkey meat, tortellini, and finely chopped parsley. Adjust soup seasoning with desired amount of kosher salt and fresh ground pepper.

To Serve

1. In a soup bowl, place 1 large ladle of garnish into center of bowl, top the bowl off with stock.
2. Drizzle with ½ tsp. extra virgin olive oil over the top of the soup.
3. Add 1 Tbsp. of grated parmigiano cheese

Nutrition:

(assumes 1 oz turkey per bowl)

- calories 338
- fat 13 grams
- saturated fat 3 grams
- cholesterol 39 mg,
- carbohydrate 37 grams
- dietary fiber 2.5 grams
- protein 19 grams.

VEGETABLE POPOVER

These vegetable popovers are excellent for individuals needing soft, easy-to-swallow foods. Eggs (or egg substitute) add an excellent source of high-quality protein. This is also a great recipe to prepare ahead of time and reheat as a healthy mini-meal.

Yield: 6 servings

INGREDIENTS

- 1 zucchini, chopped into bite-size pieces
- 1 large carrot, chopped into small pieces (about half the size of the zucchini)
- 2 tsp. olive oil
- 6 large eggs
- 1/4 cup milk (non-dairy alternative, if desired)
- 1/3 cup shredded cheddar cheese (use reduced-fat cheese for those experiencing fat intolerance)
- Salt and freshly ground black pepper, to taste
- Pinch of turmeric
- Onion powder, to taste

INSTRUCTIONS

1. Preheat the oven to 350°.
2. Spray 6 muffin cups with nonstick spray.
3. Sauté the zucchini and the carrots in 2 tsp. olive oil for 5-7 minutes.
4. In a medium bowl, whisk together the eggs and milk. Add salt, pepper, turmeric, and onion powder.
5. Distribute egg mixture evenly into muffin cups.
6. Distribute zucchini and carrots into egg mixture.
7. Bake 25 to 30 minutes, or until egg is cooked through.

NUTRITION

- calories 126
- fat 8.9 grams
- saturated fat 3.2 grams
- cholesterol 193 mg
- carbohydrate 3.4 grams
- dietary fiber 0.7 grams
- protein 8.7 grams

CHICKEN WITH QUINOA

Prepared as described this recipe will "pack a protein punch", but for additional protein add white beans and cook the quinoa in chicken broth. To add additional flavor or variety, top with low-fat sour cream and salsa for a Mexican-inspired dish. Other grains such as bulgur, rice, or couscous can also be used.

Yield: 6 servings

INGREDIENTS

- 1 Tbsp. olive oil, divided
- 1 lb. ground chicken breast
- 1 tsp. rosemary
- Pinch salt (optional)
- 1/4 tsp. pepper (optional)
- 1 cup quinoa
- 1 1/2 cups frozen kale
- 1/4 cup chicken broth

INSTRUCTIONS

1. Heat 2 tsp. olive oil in skillet; add the ground chicken, rosemary, salt, and pepper.
2. Cook until cooked through and browned.
3. Add frozen kale and chicken broth and allow to thaw and wilt; approximately 2-3 minutes.
4. While the chicken is cooking, separately cook quinoa according to package directions in medium size saucepan with remaining tsp. of olive oil. Fluff with fork when cooked.
5. Add quinoa to skillet with chicken and kale and combine well. Serve warm.

NUTRITION

- calories 217
- fat 4.8 grams
- saturated fat 0.6 grams
- cholesterol 47 mg,
- carbohydrate 19.9 grams
- dietary fiber 2.8 grams
- protein 23.9 grams

CHICKEN KEBAB WITH TZATZIKI AND PITA

A great summer time chicken recipe topped with cool, creamy tzatziki sauce. Preparation is required 2-3 hours ahead of time but well worth the extra wait time. Choose this recipe for those needing high protein, low fiber choices.

Yield: 6 servings

INGREDIENTS

Pita:

- 1 pack store-bought pita bread

Tzatziki sauce:

- 3 cucumbers
- 12 oz. plain Greek yogurt
- 1 pinch of sea salt
- 1/2 tsp. extra virgin olive oil
- 2 cloves of garlic, minced

Chicken:

- 1 1/2 pounds skinless, boneless chicken breast halves, cut into 1/2 inch pieces
- 1/4 cup olive oil for marinade
- 2 Tbsp. lemon juice
- 1 tsp. dried oregano
- 1/2 tsp. sea salt
- 6 wooden skewers

INSTRUCTIONS

Tzatziki sauce:

1. Clean and grate cucumbers. Be sure to remove seeds and peel off cucumber skin if on a low-fiber diet.
2. Strain juice and place in medium bowl.
3. Add yogurt to bowl and mix cucumbers, garlic, salt and olive oil together.
4. Cover and refrigerate for 30 minutes.

Chicken and pita:

1. Combine 1/4 cup olive oil, lemon juice, 1 tsp. oregano, and 1/2 tsp. sea salt in a large bowl.

2. Add chicken, mix with the marinade and cover the bowl.
3. Marinate in the refrigerator for at least 2 hours.
4. Skewer chicken evenly on 6 wooden skewers. Preheat grill, place pitas on grill for 2 minutes on each side until slightly browned.
5. Remove from grill and set aside.
6. Cook the skewers on the preheated grill, turning frequently until nicely browned on all sides, about 10 minutes per side. Serve with grilled pita and topped with tzatziki sauce.

NUTRITION

- calories 441
- fat 13.8 grams
- saturated fat 3 grams
- cholesterol 67 mg
- carbohydrate 44.7 grams,
- dietary fiber 3 grams
- protein 34.9 grams

CHICKEN SALAD SANDWICH

This sandwich is very easy to prepare and contains satisfying flavors and textures. It is a well-balanced meal that includes protein and carbohydrates, along with a splash of colorful fruit and herbs. For those experiencing fat intolerance, reduced fat can be substituted and walnuts can be avoided. You can also experiment with other herbs like rosemary or basil for varied flavors.

Yield: 4 sandwiches

INGREDIENTS

- 2 chicken breasts (skin on during cooking only) or approximately
- 2 cups diced or shredded cooked, skinless chicken
- 2 Tbsp. mayonnaise (may substitute yogurt - low fat or Greek - and 1 tsp. lemon juice)
- 1/4 cup sliced grapes
- 2 Tbsp. dried cranberries
- 1/4 cup chopped walnuts (optional)
- 2 tsp. dried tarragon

- 8 slices bread

INSTRUCTIONS

1. Preheat oven to 375°.
2. Roast chicken breasts for approximately 45 minutes until cooked through, juices run clear and temperature of chicken reaches 165°.
3. Remove skin from breast meat. Discard skin. Cube, dice, or shred meat.
4. Add mayonnaise, grapes, cranberries, walnuts, and tarragon.
5. Mix well and divide into 4 (~3/4 cup) portions and spread onto bread.
1. Delicious with toasted bread!

NUTRITION

- calories 237
- fat 9.8 grams,
- saturated fat 1.4 grams
- cholesterol 56 mg
- carbohydrate 13.1 grams
- dietary fiber 1.2 grams,
- protein 23.7 grams

SUMMER VEGETABLES OMELET

This omelet is an excellent source of protein and includes squash, which is generally a well-tolerated vegetable. Cheddar cheese can be substituted for another flavor of cheese, or lactose free cheese for those who are lactose intolerant.

Yield: Two 2-egg omelets

INGREDIENTS

- 2/3 cup sliced summer squash
- 2/3 cup sliced fresh zucchini
- 2 Tbsp. oil, divided
- 4 eggs, beaten, divided (may substitute 2 egg whites for each egg if needed for lower fat intake)
- 2 slices white cheddar cheese (use reduced fat cheese if experiencing fat intolerance or any flavor cheese of choice)

INSTRUCTIONS

1. Heat 1 Tbsp. oil in omelet pan over medium heat.
2. Sauté zucchini and squash in oil for 4-5 minutes until tender.
3. Remove vegetables and keep warm.
4. Add additional Tbsp. oil to warm pan. Add two beaten eggs and half of the vegetables. Flip and cook thoroughly. Fold in half and top with 1 slice of white cheddar cheese.
5. Make second omelet with remaining ingredients.

NUTRITION

- calories 310
- fat 27.4 grams
- saturated fat 9.1 grams
- cholesterol 193 mg
- carbohydrate 3.6 grams
- dietary fiber 0.8 grams
- protein 13.4 grams

SHRIMP POMODORO & ANGEL HAIR

This delicious shrimp dish provides a great source of protein, but can be substituted for chicken for those who may be allergic to shellfish. Tomato content can be reduced to a smaller quantity of diced tomato or omitted and replaced with chicken or vegetable broth in order to reduce acid content. In addition, herbs and spices can be adapted to suit flavor preferences and digestive tolerance. For those looking to add more dietary fiber, whole wheat pasta can be substituted. For those who are experiencing fat malabsorption or dairy intolerance, olive oil can be reduced and parmigiano cheese can be omitted.

Yield: 6 Servings

INGREDIENTS

- 1 lb. angel hair pasta
- 6 Tbsp. extra virgin olive oil
- 3 sprigs fresh thyme
- 8 cloves garlic (sliced paper thin)
- 3/4 cup finely chopped onion

- 1 cup tomato concasse (peeled, seeds removed, diced)
- 1 Tbsp. tomato paste
- 1/2 cup white wine (can substitute non-alcoholic cooking wine)
- 2 Tbsp. chiffonade fresh basil (stacked basil leaves, tightly rolled, thinly sliced)
- 3 Tbsp. crushed red pepper flakes (optional)
- 1 1/2 lb. size 16/20 wild shrimp
- Kosher salt (as needed)
- Fresh ground pepper (as needed)
- 1 Tbsp. minced Italian parsley
- 4 Tbsp. parmigiano cheese (optional)

DIRECTIONS FOR SAUCE:

1. In a medium sized sauce pan add 3 Tbsp. of extra virgin olive oil over medium heat and add onions. Sweat onions for 5 minutes until translucent, then add half the amount of garlic, red pepper flakes (if wanted), 2 sprigs of thyme and tomato paste.

2. Continue to cook over medium heat for 3 minutes. Add white wine (reserving 1 Tbsp. for shrimp).
3. Continue to stir and cook until wine is evaporated. Add tomato concasse, 1 tsp. kosher salt and desired amount of fresh ground pepper. Lower heat to slow simmer for 45 minutes.
4. After 45 minutes, with a hand blender, pulse to slightly puree (you do not want the sauce to be completely smooth). Pulses should be 15 2-second pulses.
5. Add parsley. Reserve for plating.

www.ingramcontent.com/pod-product-compliance
Lightning Source LLC
Chambersburg PA
CBHW070805220526
45466CB00002B/546